MEDICAL PROFESSION
PROUD TO BE A DOCTOR

DR YOGESH S. VALIMBE

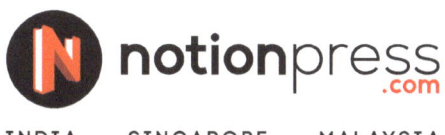

INDIA • SINGAPORE • MALAYSIA

Notion Press Media Pvt Ltd

No. 50, Chettiyar Agaram Main Road,
Vanagaram, Chennai, Tamil Nadu – 600 095

First Published by Notion Press 2021
Copyright © Dr Yogesh S. Valimbe 2021
All Rights Reserved.

ISBN 978-1-63974-644-6

This book has been published with all efforts taken to make the material error-free after the consent of the author. However, the author and the publisher do not assume and hereby disclaim any liability to any party for any loss, damage, or disruption caused by errors or omissions, whether such errors or omissions result from negligence, accident, or any other cause.

While every effort has been made to avoid any mistake or omission, this publication is being sold on the condition and understanding that neither the author nor the publishers or printers would be liable in any manner to any person by reason of any mistake or omission in this publication or for any action taken or omitted to be taken or advice rendered or accepted on the basis of this work. For any defect in printing or binding the publishers will be liable only to replace the defective copy by another copy of this work then available.

Dedicated to my beloved parents:

Late Dr. S.G. Valimbe (Father) MA, PhD (Marathi Literature)

Late Smt. Shailaja Valimbe (Mother) BA

And

My better half Smt. Sneha (Nanda) B.Sc.

Contents

Introduction 7

Chapter I	(Year 1970–1980)	9
Chapter II	(Year 1980–1990)	17
Chapter III	(Year 1990–2000)	29
Chapter IV	(Year 2000–2010)	37
Chapter V	(Year 2010–2020)	41

Introduction

Dear readers, now I am almost completing 50 years of my Medical Profession. I want to share my experience and views towards the medical profession. I am not a commercial or professional writer but an orthopaedic surgeon, Doctor. As the title of book, I am proud to be a Doctor and to be in this profession.

Book contains 5 chapters. Each chapter is about the changes in the profession starting from the year 1970. Each chapter is a story of one decade till today i.e. 2020.

Chapter I

(Year 1970–1980)

PMT is the qualifying examination for admission to the medical college. June 13th, 1970 was the date when our first PMT (Pre Medical Test) of Madhya Pradesh results were declared in all the local and National newspapers. My name also appeared in the first list of successful candidates.

PMT was started in Madhya Pradesh since 1970. Before that admissions to the Medical College were done on merit basis i.e. only on the marks obtained in Higher Secondary Certificate examination or B.Sc. FY results.

There were only six Government Medical Colleges in Madhya Pradesh. Outside candidates other than Madhya Pradesh were not allowed to appear in PMT. Total number of seats in first year Medical were only 620.

My aim to write this book is to make public and masses to be aware about this profession. It is a very Nobel profession.

Cost of treatment and medical fees of doctors are going high. I have seen medical doctors, allopathic general practitioners treating patients with just a nominal fees. Patients did have full faith on treating doctors. Doctors were just like one the family members. Bond between doctors and patients was so nice that nobody even think of abusing any doctor, even if the patient die during treatment.

Doctors – Patients relationship was very nice and doctors were also very sympathetic. There only aim was to serve humanity and save the human life.

In this book I have tried to explain, how this profession has changed and how the attitude of doctors and patients got changed.

Change is the essence of life and in my opinion it is a rule of nature.

I have divided the book in five chapters. Each chapter is story and experience of each decade starting from 1970, when I got admission to the Medical College for my first Bachelors degree of M.B.B.S. Last chapter consists of story of recent advances in medical science from 2010 to 2020.

Recently we are facing Covid 19 pandemic. My country India is doing far better than other 200 countries in the world. Richest and advanced countries like USA, Italy, Spain, Germany etc. are facing economical crises with higher mortalities from this disease.

Lastly I will write about my struggle in my life in medical profession from the year 1970 till today. I think its a story of more than fifty percent of medical graduates, who are economically middle class like me.

1970 was the year of excitement for me. As I have been admitted in M.G.M Medical College, Indore, Madhya Pradesh, my native town. First year was full of excitement, trepidations and stress of jubilation.

In the first year we had only two subjects, Anatomy (Study of normal structure of human body) and Physiology (Study of normal functioning of human body). Both the subjects were very vast, but unless you know the normal structure and function of the human body, you cannot understand disease i.e. abnormal function. You can't diagnose, investigate and treat the patient.

In the first year we had dissection of the human body i.e. Cadaver (Preserved human body), as practical in large dissection hall. It has about 30 solid marble tables and 4 to 6 students were supposed to do the dissection of different parts of human body. It was an adventure for me. Most of the students use to vomit in the early days as the dissection hall was stinking due to preservative chemical used for cadaver.

Everyone had curiosity and tremendous desire to learn. It took me more than two months to settle and acquire the acquittance with the atmosphere of the Anatomy Dissection Hall.

Many of us were disturbed due to ragging from seniors, it was a fun.

In the year 1970 President of India was Shri V.V.Giri and prime minister was Smt. Indira Gandhi.

Anwar Sodat took as the President Egypt after death of Abdul Nasser. I remember in 1972 Munich summer Olympic Games, eleven Israeli athletes were killed by five terrorist, one police personnel also died during the attack.

I used to read news paper daily and listen to the hindi filmy popular songs in Radio. I liked the programme Bianca Geet Maala from Radio Ceylon, which was broadcasted every Wednesday at 9 pm.

Those were the days when doctors were respected like God. Every parents wanted their siblings to be admitted in Medical College or Engineering College.

My elder sister, Dr. Mrs. Saroj Tapaswi, did graduation from the same college of Indore. She completed her graduation in 1967. Now practicing in Pune, Maharashtra till today. My brother-in-law is also graduate from same college and batch, Dr. Shreenivas Tapaswi. They had a big Shushrusha Hospital in Pune and had very good practice. They were busy and sometimes they worked for more then 16 hours a day. Loking to my sister, that time only I decided that I will not marry a doctor or a paramedic girl.

Medical education is a tough job. M.B.B.S. course was of four and half years. Now it is of five years. There were only three university examinations. First professional examination used to be after one and half years in which only two subjects Anatomy and Physiology were there. Now there are three subjects, Biochemistry is also added.

Second professional examination was also after one and half years. Subjects were, Pharmacology, Pathology, Preventive and Social Medicine and Forensic Medicines i.e. Juris Prudence.

This and final professional examination was also of one and half years, subjects were, 1. Surgery including Orthopaedics and ENT, 2. Medicine including Skin and Venereology, 3. Obstetrics and Gynaecology, 4. Ophthalmology.

Now they have following subjects in M.B.B.S. curriculum.

First professional after 1 year

1. Anatomy
2. Physiology
3. Biochemistry

Second professional after 2 years

1. Pharmacology
2. Pathology
3. Preventive and Social Medicine
4. Forensic Medicine

Third professional after 2 years

1. Medicine
2. Surgery
3. Obstetrics and Gynaecology
4. Ophthalmology
5. Paediatrics

(Year 1970–1980)

6. E.N.T. (Ear Nose Throat, Otorhinolaryngology)

7. Orthopaedics

8. Skin and Venereal diseases

One can do post graduation in all the above subjects. Super speciality subjects in which one can study after P.G. Degree i.e. M.S. or M.D. are

1. Cardiology

2. Neurology

3. Cardio-thoracic surgery

4. Plastic Surgery

5. Paediatric surgery

6. Neurosurgery

7. Gastroenterology

8. Nephrology

After passing M.B.B.S. one has to do one year rotating internship, they only the degree of M.B.B.S. is given to the person and only after getting the degree from University one can write Doctor infront of his/her name.

I was not a brilliant student. I used to study more during university examinations only. I got through all the examinations of M.B.B.S. in first attempt.

During the studentship my extra curricular activity (my hobby) was swimming. I was captain of my college and university swimming team. We were runner-up in the inter-university aquatic championships water polo at Jaipur in 1972 and received silver medal. We got the winner trophy in All India Inter-medical sports championships in swimming held at All India Institute Medical Sciences, New Delhi for three years consecutively.

I also represented Madhya Pradesh State in National Swimming Championships in 1973, 1974.

We had 180 students in our batch 1970 M.B.B.S. There were only 32 girls. I had good friendship with all my batchmates and it is still continuing after so many years.

I lost my father on 17th December 1969. he had suffered from from cancer of maxilla bone of chick. He was operated twice at Tata Memorial Hospital, Bombay by famous international cancer surgeon of that time Dr. Sarraiya. Later on he himself died of cancer.

My father wanted me to be a doctor. Because of his blessings only I studied and completed my M.B.B.S. course. My father late Dr. S.G. Valimbe, was Professor and head of the Department of Marathi language at Govt. Arts and Commerce College at Indore. He was M.A., Ph.D. in marathi language. During his last tenure he was Pricipal at Government Degree College, Jhabua (M.P.)

After passing the final M.B.B.S. examination in January 1975, I completed my rotating one year internship at Maharaja Yashwant Rao Hospital, Indore. Then I went to Bombay and worked for 2 years in different hospitals as House Surgeon. I worked in K.E.M. Hospital and Sir H.N. Hospital (Now it Reliance Hospital) Mumbai in Neurosurgery, Cardiovascular and Thoracic surgery and Paediatrics.

K.E.M. Hospital is the oldest and big hospital of India. It has largest OPD patients, about 5000 per day in year 1976.

I believe that, "Once you live in Bombay (Now Mumbai), you can live in any part of world."

Apart from the Medical education, the city of Mumbai, teaches you every walk of life. I learn to do hard work, humanity and sentiments from Mumbai. It is true that city of BOMBAY NEVER SLEEPS. Work is on for Mumbai 24/7. It is highly crowded city. Everyone is busy. You see the people always running here and there. Nobody has extra time to talk and relax. It is financial capital of India.

I was registered for the post graduate diploma course (D.C.H.) under late Professor Dr. S.M. Merchant at Sir H.N. Hospital. He was chief at Wadia Hospital for Children. It was a 2 years course but my ambition was to become a surgeon, so I left P.G. Course at Mumbai. I joined Madhya Pradesh Government Service in October 1977 as I was selected by P.S.C. of M.P. State.

I was posted at rural area in district Bilaspur (Now in Chattisgarh State), very remote place called Gram Faguram. It was 1200 km from my native place home town, Indore. There was no Pacca House and electricity in that village. I was the first doctor to be appointed there and remained there for 8 months, until I got transferred from that place to district place Jhabua. I worked and enjoyed at the small village Faguram having population of 5000 only. At Jhabua, I had opportunity to work as M.O. incharge of the Primary Health Centre (P.H.C.) called Ambua. It had population of 2000 only but we were covering the whole block, Alirajpur (Now it is a separate district and having population of nearly 2 lakhs.

I enjoyed the service to the poor rural people honestly. Tribes were very simple, Men used to wear only langoti to cover private parts and women a short cloth covering below waist. 90% population were uneducated. Very few schools were there in that area. One more doctor was there with me at P.H.C., Ambua. It was 200 Km away from Indore. I used to travel by bus or motor cycle, which I purchased on loan after completing my one year service.

I got married in February 1980. My better half is a science graduate. We had a Government quarter to live at P.H.C. We used to go to Alirajpur and visit our subcenters by government Jeep. Sometime my wife also accompanied and we really enjoy working and touring.

We had the facility of small operations, Immunisation of children, OPD and Postmortom of MLC cases with facility of Normal delivery cases. We used to do family planning operations also under local anaesthesia. But for Cesarian Section and some difficult cases we used to refer them to Alirajpur which was 18 KM away.

So the first decade of my medical life includes medical education and struggle for the job. After passing out from Medical College I was out of track with my college friends. There was no communication except to write letters and send them by post office.

Chapter II
(Year 1980–1990)

This decade was very important in my life and also for medical profession.

I was transferred to a remote tribe area the Jhabua district of Madhya Pradesh. I was serving poorest people of the earth.

I was blessed with two sons. One in July 1981 and second in October 1985. The Government District Hospital, Jhabua was 100 bedded newly constructed hospital. I was transferred as M.O. at District Hospital after one year in 1982. I worked sincerely and honestly till March 1985. Then I was selected to do Post graduate (M.S.) in Orthopaedic Surgery on deputation. I got admission in my old mother institute, M.G.M. Medical College, Indore (M.P.) I joined the P.G. course in 1985 January.

I met my old friends batchmates of M.B.B.S. Dr. Suredndra Lunawat, who was assistant Professor in the same college. I can't forget his help during my tenure of two years of P.G.

I passed M.S. Orthopaedics in July 1987. Then I got transferred to M.G Government District Hospital, Dewas (M.P.) The place was only 40 KM away from Indore, therefore I decided to keep my family and children at Indore for their education. Both the sons studied at prestigious school of Indore, Saint Paul's School.

When I joined at District Hospital, Dewas, there was no Orthopaedic surgeon in the Government Hospital in the whole district. Our Civil Surgeon and Chief of Hospital was very cooperative. He encouraged me to do surgeries and provided me all the instruments required. I started doing small to medium orthopaedic surgeries like plating, nailing and amputations. We used to do close reduction of fracture routinely.

Bhor Committee was formed under the Chairmanship of Mr. Bhor in 1948 for the smooth regulation of health and medical services by Government of India. the committee advised G.O.I. to form Indian Medical Services just like Indian Administrative Services (I.A.S.) but recommendation of Bhor committee were not accepted and implemented by G.O.I

Many committees were framed by G.O.I. to advise on the same subject after 1980, but not a single recommendation was accepted. It was the high time G.O.I. should have formulated our implementations because of low budget of G.O.I., it was not sanctioned.

Ttill 1990, there were only Government hospital providing health care services mainly. Only few private hospital were there.

In the capital of nation Dehli, we had only few private hospitals. They were run by the public trust Moolchand Hospital, Saint Stephen's Hospital, Hoy Family Hospital and Sir Gangaram Hospital.

That was the time when everyone including V.I.P. politicians and Beurocrates used to go to Government Hospital for treatment.

Government Hospitals were well equipped and all the facilities of treatment and operation were available in Government Hospital which provided free treatment to the poor people.

Now it is reverse, Government Hospitals lack many facilities which are provided by the rich and so called Corporate Hospitals.

Thinking of people also changed. Those who can spend money they go to private hospitals only.

In this decades there was a high population explosion in India. There was no increase in Government Hospital beds. No increase in staff.

Government Hospitals started being identified as poorly managed and less equipped centres.

With the liberation of economy in India, every thing was opened to private sector. Corporate entered in the healthcare. It became an industry. We were getting free or subsidised healthcare, we didn't realise that healthcare is an expensive affair. Our policy makers stopped investing on the technologies which were very expensive. The computer and digital era was started in our country. New technologies were imported by the big corporate hospitals.

Our landmark in the medical profession was in the year 1986. A very important judgement was passed by the full bench of 7 judges, stating that, "Medical services to the patients, for which fees was charged, will come under the preview of Consumer Protection Act (C.P.A.)

The CPA 1986 had put a curtain on the long drawn out debate between the doctors and the patients (Consumers) issue.

When the case was before the Supreme Court during 1984–1986, there was a public uproar on the kidney transplant racket. Indian Medical Association and members of M.C.I. responded about the Act. Many doctors knew that who where indulged in such practices.

This decade 1980–1990 was a milestone in the Indian Medical history. Many new researches in the medical fields were there. Many new technologies came in to the picture.

In my speciality of Orthopaedic surgery, tremendous change occurred, old knowledge, teaching and books were absolute.

We had no knowledge of C-Arm (Image Intensifier) Machine till 1987. Only portable X-Ray machine were available. There was no digital X-Ray available. By this machine we were able to take X-Ray in the operation table and can view in TV monitor. With the help of this machine orthopaedic surgeries were able to do many complicated surgeries with perfection and within very less time. Specially the trauma cases, in which fractures are to be fixed with implants like plate, screw and wires.

We learn the use of this machine and it was very helpful in orthopaedic surgery. We could see image of the X-Ray on the monitor instantly and we can also zoom image.

Medical Science progressed tremendously in this decade. Many medical centres started doing Angioplasty and Coronary bypass surgery. Many neurological patients were treated successfully by latest technology in Neurosurgery and drugs.

In Obstetrics and Gynaecology, Maternal death rate was tremendously reduced by health education to the people and latest technology to detect the congenital anomalies in the foetus by ultrasonography.

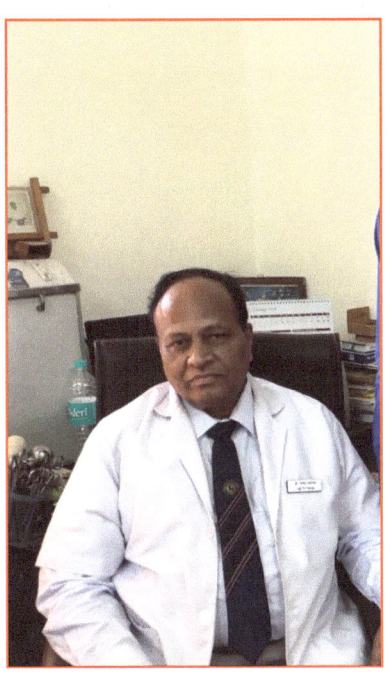

At my clinic in Dewas. M.P.

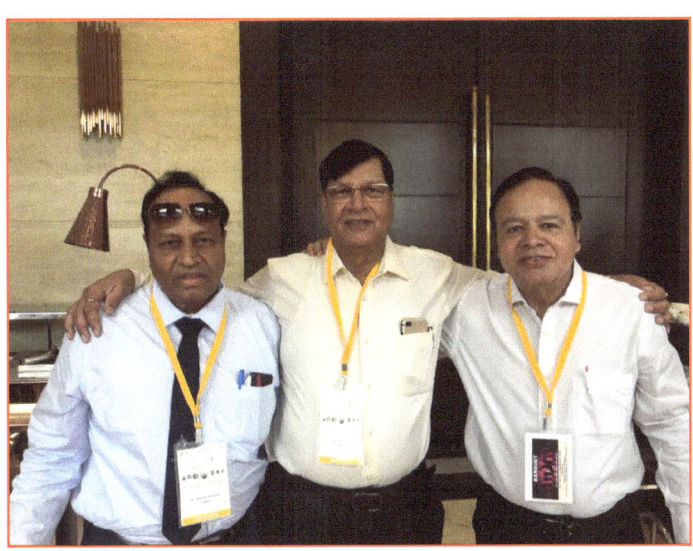

Attending conference with my friends, Ortho Surgeons and my Batchmates, L to R Myself, Dr. D.K. Jain and Professor Dr. S.K. Lunawat

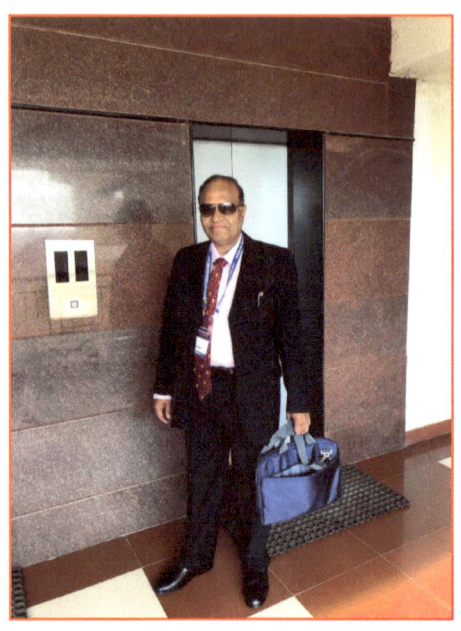

Ready to go for conference of Indian Orthopaedic Association at Bengaluru

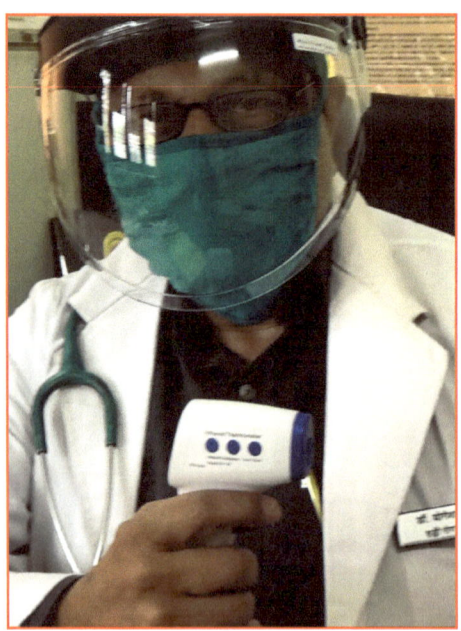

Real Corona Worrier. Practicing with all precautions

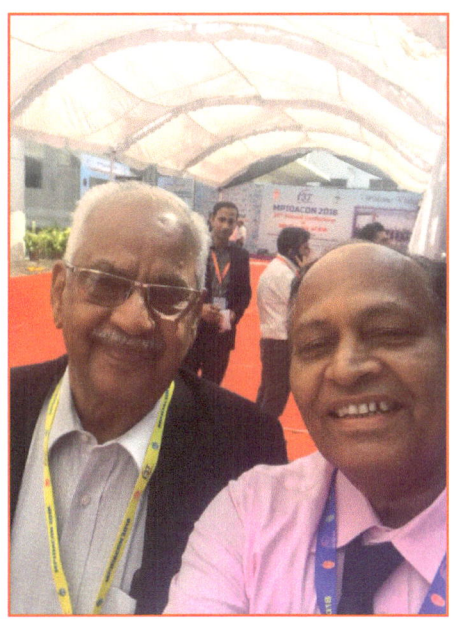

With Padamshri Dr. N.K. Laad from Mumbai, Past President of IOA

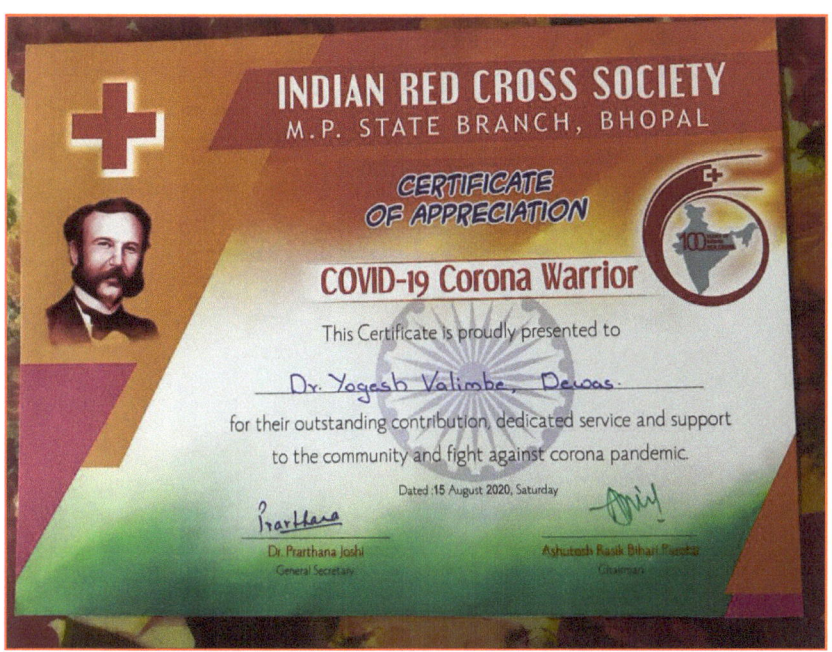

Certificate of Corona Warrier

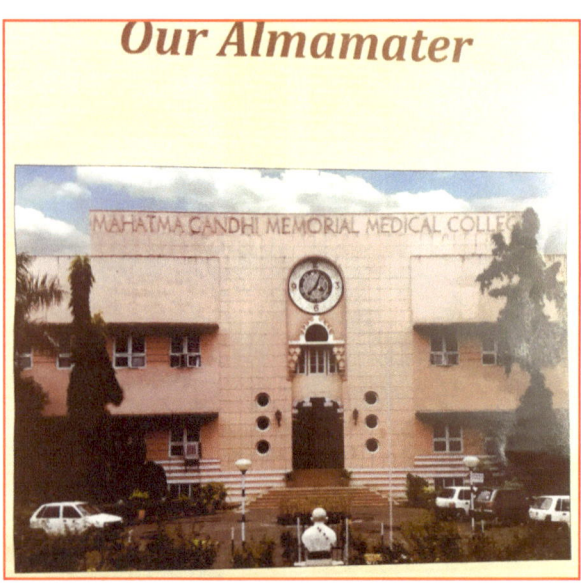

My mother institute at Indore, M.P., INDIA

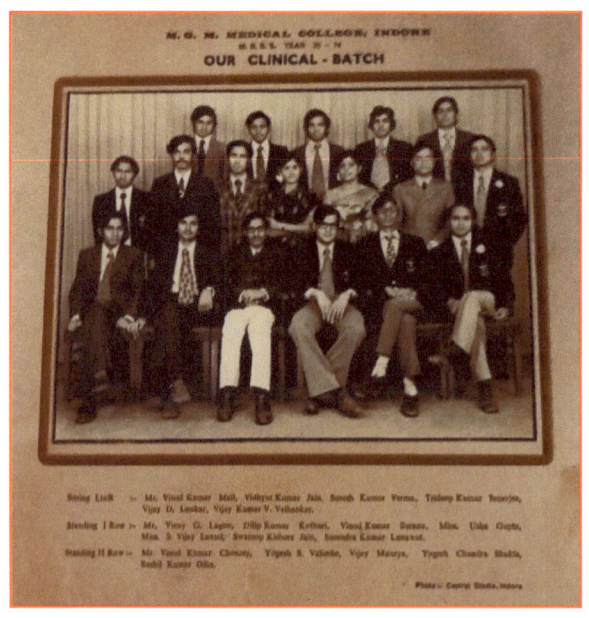

Group photo of our clinical batch. MBBS 1970-74

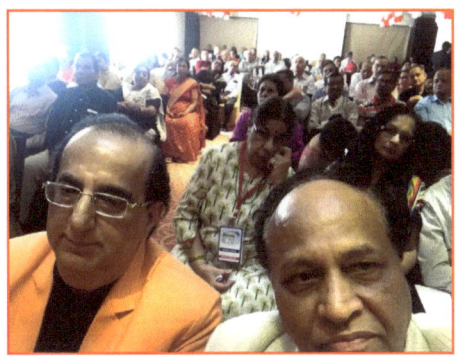

Dr. H.K. Chopra, Past President of Cardiology Society of India and my batchmate

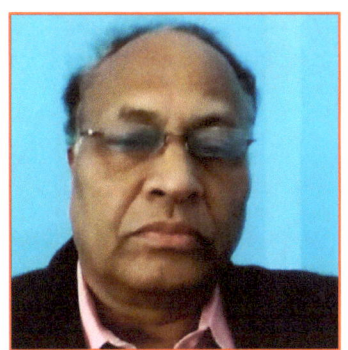

Recent photo of Myself 2021, January

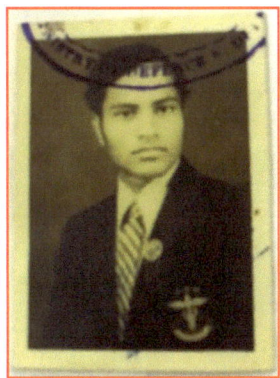

Captain of University and College Swimming team

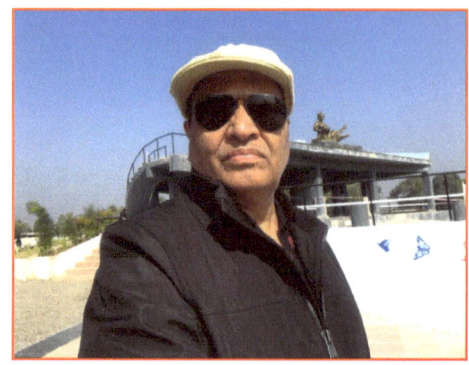

Photo at picnic

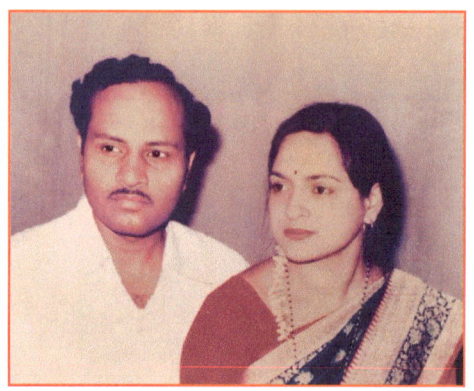

With my better half Mrs. Sneha Valimbe

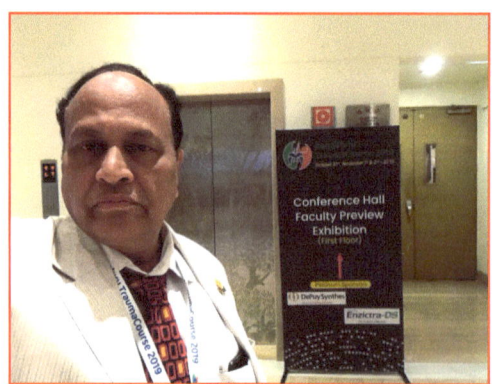

Attending Traumacourse 2019

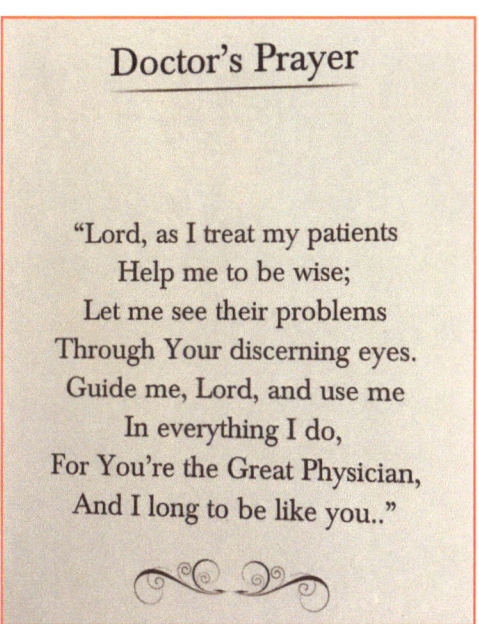

Every Doctor must remember the Prayer

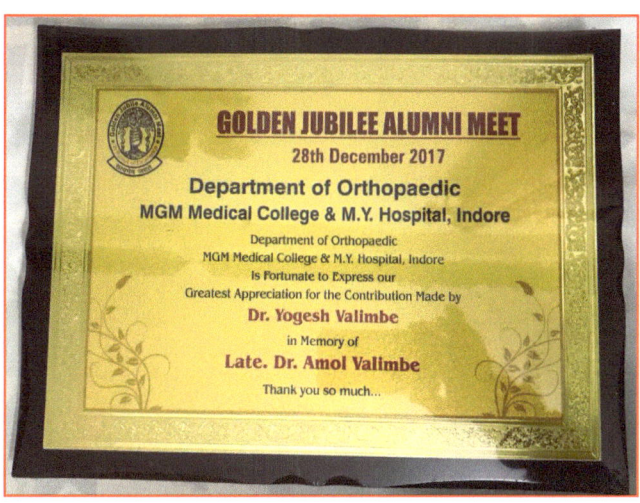

Certificate of appreciation for contributions to the Department as Alumini of my institute

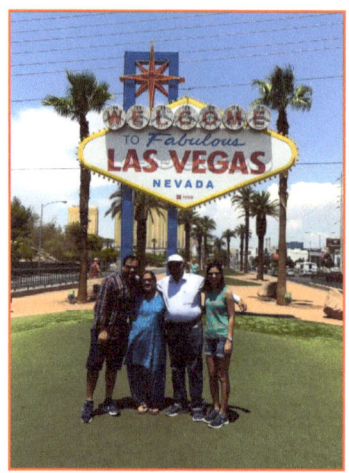
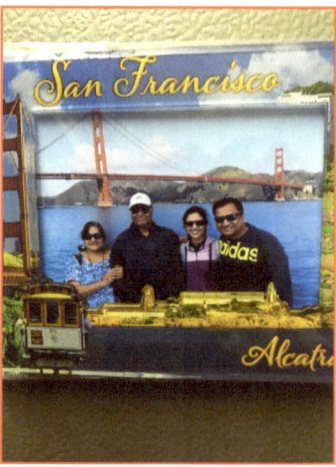
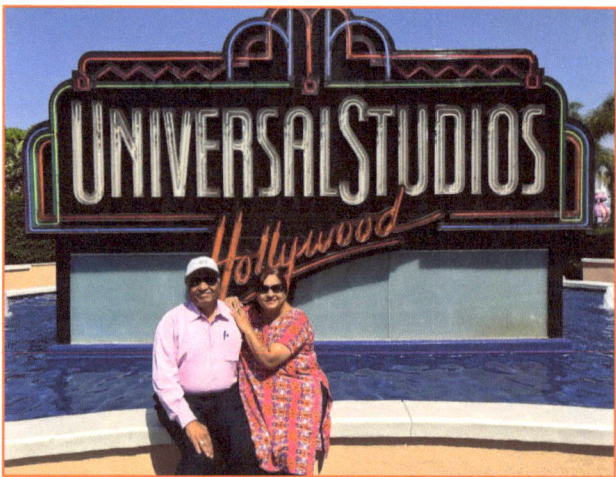
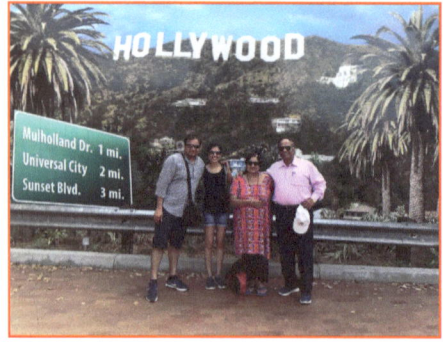
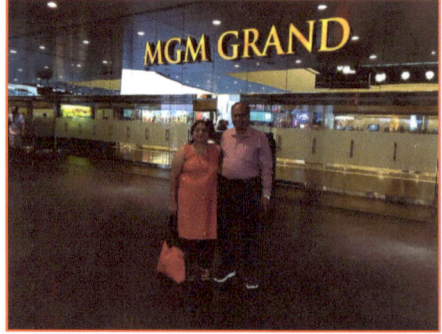

Memories of U.S.A. trip July 2017 with family

Chapter III

(Year 1990–2000)

After doing post-graduation M.S. (Master of Surgery) degree in the subject Orthopaedic Surgery, I settled in a small town near Indore, known as Dewas. It is a district place in the state of Madhya Pradesh. It has a very nice climate and the legendary classical singer respected Kumar Gandharv was residing here for his treatment of the Tuberculosis disease since long. He came here before independence and one English doctor Robert was doing his treatment. Late Padmshree Kumar Gandharv, Classical singer lived here for whole of his life.

Dewas had Five lakhs population as per 1991 census.

There are many famous temples in Dewas. Biggest temple is of Maa Chamunda Mata, which is situated on the top of a small hil in centre of the city.

Dewas is also famous for Bank Note Press of India where all denominations currency is printed.

Dewas is an industrial town and many industries are here.

Medical profession made a history in this decade year 1991 to 2000 and new advances in medical care. I was working as Medical Officer and Orthopaedic Surgeon at a small 100 beds hospital of M.P. state government. we had all the facility in all the departments for medical care.

Main Hospital was shifted in the year 1992 at new three floored large building. strength of the beds were also increased to 450 beds.

We started doing all the major and minor operations in orthopaedics, general surgery, obstetrics and gynaecology and ophthalmology.

Concept of new born care and hospital delivery came into existence in this decade only in the state of Madhya Pradesh. I.C.C.U (Intensive Cardiac Care Unit) for the heart patients and I.C.U. (Intensive Care Unit) for other emergency patient came into existence in this decade. Patients were getting highest level of care in these units.

Government of India took the project of Family Planning because of population explosion in the year 1991 census. Because the people were afraid of name family planning, specially in the young generation, the name of the department was changed as Public Health and Family Welfare Department.

Family planning programme was started again and many incentives were given to the young couples who were undergoing permanent sterilisation operation for family planning female sterilisation i.e. tube tying operation was more popular than male sterilisation operation i.e. V.T. (Vas tying) operation for male.

Family planning operations targets were fixed for the government doctors and health workers. They need to motivate the eligible couples for F.P. operations.

No political party openly supported the family planning because of the incidence in the past during Indira Gandhi's tenure in 1975, when many young male were operated by V.T. operation when they were unmarried due to strictness of Sanjay Gandhi, who was elder son of Indira Gandhi, who later died in and aeroplane accident in New Delhi.

In China family planning programme is a compulsion. Government was not giving any incentives to the second child produced but it was a crime and they would punish such couple. Because of the strictness China got over the population explosion. Their aim was "HUM DO, HAMARA EK" while in India the slogan was still "HUM DO, HAMARE DO."

As we all know in India there was a great change in countries politics and the main party Indian National Congress Party's name was changed a Indira Congress after the name of Indira Gandhi, took over as a president of the party. After her death Shri Rajeev Gandhi took over as a prime minister of India. After Rajeev Gandhi Shri P.V. Narsimha Rao was sworn as P.M. of India. That was the time when Babri Masjid was dismentalised by R.S.S. workers in Lucknow. Mr. Kalyan Sing was the Chief Minister of Uttar Pradesh State then.

We had All India Orthopaedic surgery Conference in Lucknow (U.P) in November last week in 1992. I visited personally and saw Ramlala Temple and Babri Masjid. That time people of Ayodhya and U.P. were talking about the demolition of Babri Masjid on 4th December 1992.

I myself presented a research paper in Lucknow Conference. Subject was on my Thesis Topic during my P.G. "Evaluation of Results of Prosthetic Replacement in Femoral Neck Fracture." I prepared the paper under my reverend teacher professor Dr. S.K.Ohari. He was a divine soul. I still remember his dynamic teachings and surgery.

Professor Dr. D.K.Taneja was also my guide and he has helped me in all walks of life.

I sincerely thank my teachers during P.G. at M.G.M. Medical College, Indore. They were Late Professor Dr. S.K.Ohari, M.S.D. Ortho, H.O.D Department of orthopaedic surgery, late Professor Dr. V.S.Inamdar, Professor Dr. D.K.Taneja. Professor Dr. P.K.Bhargaw, Professor Dr. S.K.Lunawat.

Dr. S.K.Lunawat my batchmate during M.B.B.S. in the same college. He was lecturer when I did my P.G. Dr. Taneja, Dr. V.S.Inamdar were at the post of Reader, while Dr. P.K.Bhargav was also lecturer at the same time.

I was doing M/P.Government service at District Hospital, Dewas. We were allowed to do private practice. I used to operate my private patient at Kareem Nursing Home, Dr. W.R.Gajdhar, M.S. (General Surgery) was owner of the hospital.

We purchased a C-Arm (Image Intensifier Machine) in partnership. It was a first C-Arm machine in Dewas.

I was leading Orthopaedic Surgeon in Dewas district and we used to operated all the minor and major surgeries. In the year 1995 I purchased a new Maruti car. I travelled in the car with my family and kids widely. Long tours were made at Mumbai and Pune. I used to live with my mother at Dewas and my wife used to live in Indore because of the education of our children. Both sons were studying in prestigious Saint Paul's School, Indore.

I did purchased a flat at Indore in old palacia.

This decision was very important for my life as I grew both my health and wealth.

We were completing 25 years of our admission in M.G.M. Medical College, Indore for M.B.B.S. in1995. Some of the batchmate in Indore organised a reunion programme of our batchmates. Preparation were started in 1995 from searching names and addresses, phone numbers of batchmates. It was given a very nice name SIJUCEL 1995.

The Long form of it was Silver Jubilee Union Celebration. More then 120 batchmates were present on this occasion. We enjoyed it, our old friends and most of friends came with their family and spouses. It was held at our mother institute M.G.M. Medical College, Indore auditorium. One day was reserved for outdoor activities and we enjoyed it as a picnic at Rau.Hotel Mashal. That was the whole day programme an all enjoyed with family. There was a nice water park and we enjoyed the various slides in the water park.

In the year 1997 my elder son Amol cleared All India P.M.T. with good marks. He got admission in Seth G.S. Medical College, Mumbai, which

(Year 1990–2000)

is attached to famous K.E.M. Hospital. Its a prestigious college and it ranked amongst the top 10 Medical Colleges in India.

In this decades number of General Practitioners i.e. M.B.B.S. doctors is redused and every Medical Graduate wanted to do post graduate degree.

In my opinion there was a lot of difference in income of Specialist and G.P. Specialist doctors were earning more than double to that of G.P. Some of the specialist who were the top in their field were earning more the double than their junior counterparts.

Money is required by everyone for food, shelter and for the family. But it is not everything. After some earning one wants a good respectable position in the society.

Medical profession is a noble profession and in our branch many patients remember you for their whole life. They feel obliged. Many of our patients treat doctors next to God.

In this decade I was doing general duty of a medical officer as I was not promoted as a class one specialist post. many times when I was doing emergency night duties of government hospital, different types of serious cases used to come and we had to manage them.

Sometimes we had to face the anger of the patient's relatives who died.

All the private hospitals and nursing home used to refer serious patients to Government Hospital during that time in the night. So that the mortality rate were much more in Government Hospital.

Many times we have to give explanation for the young patient death during the death audit meeting.

I used to attend all India and state conference of Orthopaedic Associations every year since 1991. We gain knowledge of the subjects and the recent advances which have come up in the field of surgery.

Because of these conferences we could travel to different cities of India. Many workshops and C.M.E. (Continuous Medical Education were held regularly.

I attended many of them and they help me in my profession. I could do many difficult surgeries after attending the workshops and conferences.

I could visit many big cities like New Delhi, Mumbai, Kolkata, Chennai, Bengaluru, Lucknow, Hyderabad, Mysore, Ahmedabad, Jaipur. In Madhya Pradesh also Conference of Indian Orthopaedic Association was held in Indore, Bhopal, Jabalpur and Gwalior.

In our Government set up we had the following posts for 500 bedded district hospital.

1. One post of Chief Medical and Health Officer, CHMO, who was responsible for the health care of the whole district.
2. One post of Civil Surgeon cum Chief Hospital Superintended, he was overall incharge of the main hospital and was responsible for all health care of urban population.
3. Class I specialists. We had Medical Specialist – 4 Posts, Surgical Specialist – 4 Posts, Obstetrics and Gynaecologist – 4 posts, Paediatrician – 4 posts, Ophthalmologist, Orthopaedician and ENT specialist – 2 posts each, Pathologist – 2 posts, Radiologist – 1 post.
4. Class II PGMO – 10 posts, and
5. General duty Medical Officers – 10 posts.

Class II MO were also gazetted officer. They were doing general duty in emergency. They have to perform post-mortem by rotation duties. I was also PGMO, and I did work in Orthopaedic Surgery Department. I used to do general duties also. We had to deal the medicolwegal cases also like poisoning, accident cases or assault cases. we had to record their findings and treatment and many times had to attend session and magistrate courts a an expert witness.

We had to work for the all national health programmes. We had to issue different medical certificates to people for leave purpose. Every district has a District Medical Board and I was the member and incharge of District Orthopaedic Medical Board. We had to examine the orthopedically handicapped person and give them certificate with percentage of disability.

Sometimes we have to perform family planning surgeries and many times we have to attend camp at different P.H.C.s. We have to attend Orthopaedic Handicapped Camp every year at every Tehsil or Block level.

When I look back and remember the old days of 1991 to 2000, when I was 40 years of age, I enjoyed working with enthusiasm. at this age I think every doctor must be busy, working for 24*7.

Government Medical Officer has to do multiple duties and I don't remember that I had taken any long leave of more than a week in this decade. Really I am proud that I am a doctor and I really enjoyed working for patients, Nation and of course for family.

Chapter IV

(Year 2000–2010)

Starting of this decade with a blow for the people of Gujrat state in our country on 26th January 2001, when the whole nation was busy in celebrating the 52nd Republic day, there was a severe earthquake in Kutch and Bhuj, at about 8:45 AM. This earthquake was at very high magnitude of 7.7 Mw on Richter scale and it lasted for 101 seconds. It was spread over nearly 16 KMs in the residential area and within a minute the whole area and city was dismantled. Many high building were flat on the Earth. About 20,000 people died and millions were injured.

Gujrat Chief minister invited medical teams with doctors from all the neighbouring states to help and manage the disaster. As there were millions of people injured and it took one week to manage the injured people. I had an opportunity to work for the humanity and I voluntarily gave my name to be included in the team. CMHO Dewas sent a team of 8 doctors to Gujrat for working. We reached Ahamdabad and contacted Collector there, who sent our team to Palanpur where doctors are required for the help of local doctors. A big government hospital about 500 bedded was converted into disaster management hospital and all the facilities were given by the government to needy injured persons. Many injured persons were brought from Bhuj where the earthquake occurred. We took care of injured persons with local doctors. Coincidentally CMHO of Palnpur was my batchmate, Dr. Rajendra Nagdawho helped us like a brother and praise our work. We did many orthopaedic operation like plating, nailing etc. for many patients. I was lucky to serve the needy people of Gujrat State.We were felicitated by local Lions Club of Palanpur and

Collector of Palanpur gave us very nice certificate of appreciation for the service of injured.

I can't forget the time. I myself realised the importance of medical profession at that time. as per Hippocratic Oth we were serving injured persons without considering their cast and religion. Really we are proud to be doctors and almighty God gave us an opportunity to serve the needy persons.

Many doctors of Dewas wanted to go Gujrat and serve people there but they couldn't go due to restrictions.

This decision was very important for my life. In the year 2002 my elder son completed his M.B.B.S. from K.E.M., Mumbai. He wanted to do P.G. in orthopaedic surgery. He passed Pre P.G. All India NEET examination with good rank. He was given admission to the G.R.M.C., Gwalior for P.G. in Orthopaedic Surgery which he completed in 2005. He got married with Medico girl, who completed her M.B.B.S. from G.R.M.C., Gwalior. They were blessed with a daughter. He worked in Mumbai for one year and then joined Aurbindo Medical College, Indore as Assistant Professor in Department of Orthopaedics. During this period my daughter in law completed her M.B.A. in Hospital Management from University of Indore.

I got promotion in the Government service and became class I orthopaedic specialist in 2008 August. During this decade my wealth improved. I built home in 2001 at Dewas and decided to live permanently in Dewas.

In the year 2007, I was transferred to a small village at Khargone District, due to politics but didn't go and managed to cancel the order.

There were so many workshops, conferences in all the subjects throughout the years. Doctors gained knowledge and they knew about the recent advances in each subject. Quality of treatment was increased and many diseases were treated successfully which were having no treatment, such as most of the cancers, heart diseases, blood diseases were cured successfully.

If I say that medical science has gone up to level where only a dead person can't be made alive.

Longevity of person increased and in India the average life expectancy is about 70 years.

Because of the availability of safe drinking water, many water born diseases were controlled. Health facilities to the poorest people are available free of charge in Government Hospitals. Health education was given to the people by the government officials and N.G.O.s.

Due to better immunisation schedule, the infant mortality was reduced tremendously in this decade.

Chapter V
(Year 2010–2020)

In this decade many ups and downs came in my life. this decade will be remembered for the development of India. Many large roads were built on the basis of Public-Private Partnership.

Indian railway also completed Konkan Route from Mumbai to Goa. Indian railway also expected its track upto Shrinagar in the North. Previously it was upto Jammu only.

My younger son completed his graduation from Manipal University in Engineering and got job in Bangalore. He went to U.S.A. for the project of the company.

We were blessed with granddaughter and all time enjoyed with her activites.

On 24th March 2012, W.H.O. declared our India as free from the dreadful disease called Poliomyelitis. After that not a single case was recorded of Poliomyelitis in our country. There were huge number of people who suffered from the disease poliomyelitis in childhood and many have weakness in legs, known as post polio paresis. There is no sensory loss but muscles of the lower limbs become weak and they are permanently weak due to which limbs become deformed and many persons have difficulty in walking, standing.

I was member of the District Medical Board and we used to give certificates to the orthopedically handicapped persons with percentage of disability. Certificate was necessary for many government schemes. Sometimes certificate was needed for the road traffic accidents claim in the court of law.

One tragic incidence occurred on 13th June 2012. My elder son Dr. Amol, who was also an Orthopaedic surgeon met with a fatal road accident while he was coming back to Indore from Shirdi. He was travelling with his wife by his car. Driver was driving the car and his car struck with the truck.

I was regularly attending the conferences of Indian Orthopaedic Association and Madhya Pradesh State Orthopaedic Association. The workshops in the conferences were very helpful in learning the various procedures and the major operations. We also get recent knowledge of the subject. Every member of the association can take part in the conference. He can read his selected research papers. He can ask his difficulties to the faculty or speaker. I always attend the conference with my spouse and some conferences with my son. I enjoyed sightseeing, entertainment and cultural programmes during the conferences.

We enjoyed our trip to Jammu and Kashmir in 2011 with our group of doctor friends. Natural beauty of Shrinagar was really wonderful. It is called as Switzerland of India (I think Kajjiyar of Himachal Pradesh is also called as Switzerland of India) *Some Indian call it Dharti Ka Swarg.*

I got retirement from the state government services in April 2017 after a long 40 years of service.

My younger son Anop was in New Jersey, USA. He arranged our trip to USA. We enjoyed the trip as our daughter in law Ankita was also there. USA is a vast country. There is time difference of 3 hours from east coast, New York city to west coast, California or Los Angels. We were there for a more then a month. We visited many places including New York City, Nigeria falls, Washington DC, Los Angels, Las Vegas, Hollywood, California, Golden Gate etc. USA trip was in month of July 2017.

After retirement from Government service on 30th April 2017, I am feeling very much relaxed. I started many charitable activities. I joined senior citizen's club I see them free of charge at my residence on every tuesday and Saturday at their office from 4 PM to 6 PM. I again joined Lion's Club of Dewas City. I was a charter member of this club which started in 1997. I was elected as President of Indian Medical Association, Dewas Branch. In my opinion a doctor in the society does maximum charity in comparison to others. You can't count doctor's charity in terms of money.

Government doctors do more charity than private. They were always overburdened. Previously government doctors were more respected than private doctors but now private doctors are more respected and praised than government doctors.

I am proud to be a doctor because:

1. It's a noble profession.
2. They are respected in every society.
3. God has given the power to treat and cure the patients suffering from the diseases.
4. Doctors have not to worry of their bread and butter.
5. A doctor can do a lot of charity.
6. He is supposed to be a next to God by many.

CORONA COVID-19

A new virus and disease came in to existence from January 2020, origin is supposed to be from Wuhan city, China.

It is spreading all over the world. WHO has declared it as Pandemic. Millions of death have occurred due to this disease.

There were many strains of Corona virus were present before but this Covid-19 strain was very dangerous. Many people in world succumb to death due to it. It is supposed to be highly infectious and it spreads by droplet infection.

No drug is 100 percent effective against this virus. Mortality rate is very high in many developed countries like USA, France, Italy, Germany, China. But now mortality rate is redusing.

In India Covid-19 infection came in the month of March 2020. For the first time lockdown was announced by the Prime Minister of India on 24th March 2020. He advised people to wear mask and follow social distancing. It is claimed that we have saved more than 70000 lives due to timely taken actions like lock down etc.

Health department advised to use sanitisers, and repeated hand washing by any soap.

All the Malls, shops and public transport were closed and even the examination of board were abandoned.

Everybody was advised to stay at home or where ever he was. All International and National Flights were cancelled. Indian railways were also stopped for the passengers. Only goods trains and transport vehicles were allowed to run. All the Government Hospitals were made ready and equipped for the outbreak of the disease Covid-19.

WHO declared it pandemic i.e. the disease is spread globally.

All the factories and non-essential services, even the many government offices were closed for some period in lockdown.

As the disease was new, many health workers and doctors died due to it. Many scientists, doctors and pathologist worked day and night for the invention of prophylaxis of diease by immunisation and vaccine for the disease.

Main symptoms of the disease were dry cough, cold and fever, followed by difficulty in breathing. Most vulnerable population was old age people more than 70 years of age. Persons having high blood pressure, diabetes, heart disease or kidney or liver diseases were also warned to be more careful. as the mortality was more due to Covid-19 with these diseases.

Separate isolation wards with ICCU (Intensive Cardiac care Unit) were established for the critical care of the patients having this disease. Many patients needed ventilators because of difficulty of breathing and low oxygen saturation in their lungs.

The disease was diagnosed by throat and nasopharyngeal swab. All the persons were admitted and treated in hospitals having facilities of treatment of Covid-19. In many cities separate Covid Hospitals were established to treat these patients. Every case was taken to stop the spread of infection and disease. Even the dead bodies of person died due to corona were packed in special 3 layers of cloth and disposed as per the direction of Government.

Many suspected patient having symptoms of the Corona was taken care immediately and his sample was taken for investigation from throat and nose swab.

Number of laboratories were increased for the diagnosed of the disease.

HOW THE SCENARIO AND CONCEPTS OF COVID-19 HAS CHANGED FROM BEGINNING TILL TODAY:- We observed –

1. Covid-19 was considered first to cause viral pneumonia, but now it is understood to be a mysterious virus and unpredictable.
2. It does't attack joints or larynx, so no joint involvement or hoarseness of voice.
3. No lymph nodes involvement.

4. Previously considered as non-inflammatory, but now it's considered inflammatory.

5. Disease was considered critical on anyday previously but now days 3–6 are considered to be critical.

6. Social distancing has changed person to person, physical distancing.

7. Surface to human transmission (Micro-droplets) was mostly considered as a rout of transmission nut now micro droplet in air.

8. Wearing mask in public made compulsory.

9. Distancing of 3 feet has changed to 6 feet. With micro-droplets this distance is 9 feet.

10. Earlier very high mortality (10%), recused to 0.3%

11. In early days no specific drugs were available but now it the inflammatory parameters are raised then steroids and dediwevs raised then anticoagulants given with antiviral drugs.

12. Earlier when it first begin in Wuhan, China it was considered as pulmonary Covid (lung disease) and CT diagnosed was necessary but now it is also recognised as non-inflammatory Covid, involving GIT and CNS (Gut and Brain)

13. Previously typical fever at the time of presentation but now no fever at presentation.

14. No loss of smell and taste has been in 20–30 % of patient's, disease is mild in nature.

I became doctor on 15th March 1976, when I got MBBS degree from University of Indore and on 17th March 1976. I was legally allowed to practice medicine, write prescription and examine patients when I was registered as medical practitioner with the Mahakaushal

Medical Council, Indore. My registration number is 5681. Since them I am practicing as medical doctor for more then 45 years. I did post graduation MS (Orthopaedics surgery) in 1987 from my parent institute MGM Medical College, Indore and Devi Ahilya Vishvavidyalay, Indore.

I am proud to be a doctor, though my field is not to treat Corona patients, but as a doctor I have full knowledge of the disease Corona and I am helpful to the society because of my study and I can teach people about the disease and therefore I am proud that I am of some help to the society in this pandemic.

www.ingramcontent.com/pod-product-compliance
Lightning Source LLC
Chambersburg PA
CBHW041206180526
45172CB00006B/1209